Healthy Healing
Library Series
by
Linda Rector-Page, N.D., Ph.D

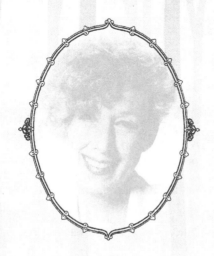

Body Cleansing
&
Detoxification To
Fight Disease

The
Healthy Healing
Library Series

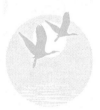

As affordable health care in America becomes more difficult to finance and obtain, more attention is being focused on natural therapies and healthy preventive nutrition. Over 65% of Americans now use some form of alternative health care, from vitamins to massage therapy to herbal supplements. Everyone wants and needs more information about these methods in order to make informed choices for their own health and that of their families.

Herbal medicines are especially in the forefront of modern science today because they have the proven value of ancient wisdom and a safety record of centuries..

The Healthy Healing Library Series

ISBN:1-884334-06-7

Published by Healthy Healing Publications, Inc.
16060 Via Este,
Sonora, Ca., 95370.

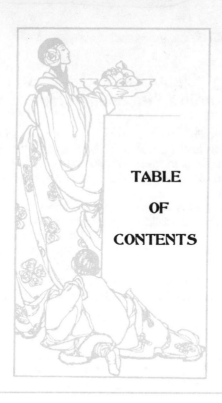

TABLE

OF

CONTENTS

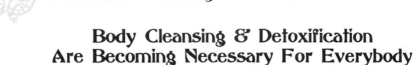
Body Cleansing & Detoxification Are Becoming Necessary For Everybody

Environmental toxins, secondary smoke, caffeine and alcohol overload, prescription and pleasure drug abuse, "hidden" chemicals, pollutants and pesticides in foods causing allergies and addictions, not to mention cumulative daily stress are all becoming an increasing part of our lives. **There is no doubt about it.** We are immersed in synthetic substances. More than 2 million are known, 25,000 are added **each year,** and over 30,000 are being produced on a commercial scale. Only a tiny fraction are ever tested for toxicity. Some of the most threatening include:

- Toxic lead in our air, dust and drinking water
- Carbon monoxide, concentrated in cigarette smoke and high combustion engine areas
- Industrial waste and corroded plumbing leach into and pollute ground water
- Carcinogenic PAHs (polynuclear aromatic hydrocarbons), formed from burning substances such as coal and tobacco. (Cigarette smoke also prevents cilia protective projections from sweeping pollutants out of the lungs.)
- Hexavalent chromium linked to gastrointestinal hemorrhage and cancer, found in the air, cigarette smoke and water
- Radioactive metals released as fly ash from power plants that accumulate in our bones.

Because the molecular structure of most chemical carcinogens interacts with DNA, long term exposure to pollutants can result in metabolic and genetic alteration that affects cell growth, behavior and immune response. The newest testing by the World Health Organization implicates toxic environmental chemicals in 60 to 80 percent of all cancers. Tests also link pesticides and pollutants to birth defects, still births and now breast cancer. **The wide variety of toxic substances means that every system of the body is affected - from the deep level tissue damage to sensory deterioration.**

When the saturation of toxic matter in the tissues, and the lack of anti-oxidants and minerals in vital body fluids occurs, immune defenses are thrown out of balance, vitality is reduced, and eventually disease results. Circumstances like this have become the prime factor in today's "civilization" diseases, such as Candida Albicans, Chronic Fatigue Syndrome (EBV), Cancer, Lupus, and even AIDS.

Chemical oxidation is the other process that affects body degeneration and allows disease. The oxygen that "rusts" and ages us also triggers free radical activity. Free radicals are incomplete molecules that attach and take parts of other molecules causing damage to DNA and other cell components. If you didn't have a reason to reduce your fat intake before, oxygen combines with fats in our cells to speed up the free radical deterioration process.

How can we remain healthy in a destructive environment?

First, while most of us can't escape to a remote, pristine habitat, we can take a closer look at our own air, water and food, and keep it as clean as possible. Second, we can take positive steps to keep the body's own self-cleansing systems in good working order, so that toxins are eliminated quickly.

In the past, detoxification was used either clinically for recovering alcoholics and drug addicts, or individually as a once-a-year mild "spring cleaning" for general health maintenance. Today, because we are surrounded by increasing involuntary toxicity, detoxification is becoming more necessary not only for health, but for the quality of our lives. Optimally, one should seriously cleanse the body twice a year, especially in the spring, summer or early fall, when sunlight and natural vitamin D offer the body an extra boost.

Herbs are effective for a broad spectrum of body cleansing goals.

Herbs, particularly organically grown herbs, are rich in food-source minerals, vitamins, amino acids, and enzyme precursors. In the dried state, herbs provide concentrated, whole food nutrition that becomes part of the body to stimulate cleansing, fuel regrowth, and build resistance to disease. Herbs are unique among therapeutic media in these abilities, in a way that drugs, or even partitioned substances like vitamins are not. They work **with** the body's own action as a source of life and growth. This is the key to their success as natural medicines.

A good detox program should be in three stages:
❋Cleansing ❋Rebuilding ❋Maintaining

**Herbs, in their abundance of diversity
and in the specific nature of their activity
are optimally suited to these tasks.**

BLOOD CLEANSING

While the body has its own self-purifying complex for maintaining a healthy "river of life", the best way to protect yourself from disease is to keep those cleansing systems in good working order. Although not immediately obvious, toxins ingested in sub-lethal amounts often eventually add up to disease-causing amounts. Slow viruses leading to such nerve diseases as M.S. can enter the cells and remain dormant for years, mutating and feeding on toxic substances, then reappear in a more dangerous form than they entered. This is especially true in the three blood cleansing systems: the liver, the kidneys and the lymph glands. The best way to begin a deep body cleanse is to focus on those three areas.

Many people start a cleanse with a short 3 to 7 day juice fast to release toxins from the body more quickly. A cleansing diet may be used before and during any natural therapeutic program, unless you are very weak or highly toxic. A person with exceedingly low energy will be weakened too much by heavy elimination; a cleansing diet undertaken with a highly toxic system tends to drive the poisons into the bloodstream too fast, causing unnecessary overload reactions.
See "COOKING FOR HEALTHY HEALING" by Linda Rector-Page for full, detailed cleansing diets.

Herbs can also provide strengthening support for a successful blood cleanse. Detoxifying herbs can maintain energy levels and nerve stability during heavy metabolic waste elimination. A good example of a cleansing and purifying herbal tea with this type of activity might look like this:
RED CLOVER, HAWTHORN LF. & FLWR., ALFALFA LF., NETTLES, SAGE, HORSETAIL HERB, ECHINACEA, MILK THISTLE SD., PAU D'ARCO, GOTU KOLA, LEMON GRASS, BLUE MALVA, YERBA SANTA.

Herbs can supply concentrated chlorophyll benefits and alkalize body acidity. The molecular composition of chlorophyll is so close to that of human haemoglobin that a series of green drinks is almost like giving yourself a small, purifying transfusion.
An herbal green drink with energizing properties looks like this:
BARLEY GRASS PWD., ALFALFA, BEE POLLEN, APPLE PECTIN, CHLORELLA, SIBERIAN GINSENG, ACEROLA CHERRY, SARSAPARILLA, DULSE, DANDELION LF., GOTU KOLA, LICORICE, DANDELION RT., OAT FLOUR, LEMON JUICE PWD., IN A BASE OF WHOLE RICE PROTEIN.

A serious blood cleansing program should be accompanied by a raw vegetable and fruit juice-based diet. Vegetable and fruit juices stimulate rapid and heavy waste elimination, a process that often generates mild symptoms of a "healing crisis". A slight headache, nausea, bad breath, body odor and dark urine occur as the body accelerates release of accumulated toxins. A daily dosage of 5 to 10,000mg. of ascorbate Vitamin C is recommended during serious cleansing, to help keep the body alkaline, encourage oxygen uptake, and promote collagen development for new healthy tissue. Vitamin C should be added especially if you are detoxifying from alcohol or drug overload.

An effectivel herbal formula for blood cleansing might look like this: **RED CLOVER, LICORICE, ASCORBATE VIT.C 50MG, PAU D'ARCO, ECHINACEA RT., GOLDENSEAL RT., SARSAPARILLA, BURDOCK RT., ALFALFA, KELP, AMERICAN GINSENG, GARLIC, BUTTERNUT, MILK THISTLE, PORIA MUSHROOM, DANDELION, ASTRAGALUS, YELLOW DOCK, BUCKTHORN, PRICKLY ASH BK.**

As noted earlier, **heavy metal poisoning** has become a major health problem of modern society. Numerous studies indicate a strong relationship between heavy metal storage in the body, childhood learning disabilities and criminal behavior. If you served in Vietnam, if your work puts you in contact with petro-chemicals or solvents, if you live near a congested highway, or in a crop-dusting fly-way, check yourself for the following symptoms of heavy metal/chemical toxicity:

1) **a deep, choking cough**
2) **depression, memory loss and unusual insomnia**
3) **schizophrenic behavior, seizures, periodic black-outs**
4) **sexual dysfunction**
5) **black spots on the gum line; bad breath/body odor**
6) **loss of hand/eye coordination, especially in driving**
7) **unusual, severe reactions to foods and odors**

Do not go on an all-liquid diet when trying to release heavy metals or chemicals from the body. They enter the bloodstream too fast and heavily for the body to handle, and will poison you even more.

Do include daily in your diet: brown rice, miso soup. a glass of aloe vera juice and a glass of fresh carrot juice. Include artichokes to promote the flow of bile, the major pathway for chemical release from the liver. High sulphur foods like garlic, onions and beans are important. Other foods should be organically grown as much as possible.

An effective herbal remedy course should include **ECHINACEA ROOT 100% EXTRACT or PAU DE ARCO/ECHINACEA EXTRACT,** 2 to 3 times daily, a green herb supplement such as **spirulina** in a drink or tablets, and the following compound to help neutralize and release hazardous chemicals:
ASCORBATE VIT. C, BLADDERWRACK, KELP, BUGLEWEED, ASTRAGALUS, PRICKLY ASH BK., LICORICE, PARSLEY RT., POTASSIUM CHL. 25MG.

After a serious blood cleanse, an herbal combination to stimulate better circulation, to deter formation and "stickiness" of serum lipids and to maintain arterial blood composition would be recommended. The following formula is particularly effective when circulation is sluggish or impeded, and vascular tone is weak. It is rich in absorbable herbal iron. Many people report a tingle in the hands and feet after using this tea as circulation increases to the extremeties.
HAWTHORNE LF. & FLWR., BILBERRIES, KUKICHA TWIG, GINGER, HEARTSEASE, GINKGO BILOBA, PAU D'ARCO, RED SAGE, LICORICE, WHITE SAGE, CALENDULA FLWR., YELLOW DOCK, PEPPERMINT, ASTRAGALUS.

A strong, accompanying supplement program should include protective anti-oxidants such as pycnogenol, co-enzyme Q10, beta-carotene, vitamin C (5 to 10,000mg. daily), and cysteine, a heavy metal chelator.

LIVER CLEANSING

An effectiive liver cleanse is an integrated support function for clean blood. The health and vitality of the body depend to a large extent on the health and vitality of the liver. Blood flows directly from the gastrointestinal tract to the liver, so it can neutralize or alter some of the toxic substances before they are distributed to the rest of the body through the blood. Blood also **keeps returning to the liver,** processing toxins again and again so that most are altered by the time they are excreted by the bile or kidneys. Obviously it makes good sense to keep your liver in good working order.

The liver can deal with a wide range of toxic chemicals, drugs, alcohol, solvents, formaldehyde, pesticides and food additives. It is the body's most complex organ - a powerful chemical plant that converts everything we eat, breathe and absorb through the skin into life-sustaining substances. The liver is a major blood reservoir, forming and storing red blood cells, and filtering toxins at a rate of a quart of blood per minute. A healthy liver produces natural antihistamines to keep immunity high. It manufactures bile to digest fats, excrete cholesterol, aid digestion and prevent constipation. It metabolizes proteins and carbohydrates, and secretes hormones and enzymes. It is a vast storehouse for vitamins, minerals, and enzymes, and secretes them as needed to build and maintain healthy cells.

With the acknowledgement that most of us are continually assailed by toxins in our food, water and air, it is generally realized that none of us has a truly healthy liver. **The good news is that the liver has amazing rejuvenative powers, and can continue to function when as many as 80% of its cells are damaged.** Even more remarkable, it regenerates its own damaged tissue.

Be good to your liver!

I recommend a short liver cleanse and detoxification twice a year in the spring and fall to maximize its abilities, using the extra vitamin D from the sun to help. If your liver is seriously toxic, a complete liver renewal program can take from three to six months.

Some watchwords for liver health:

➝ Good liver function is dependent on the amount and quality of oxygen coming into the lungs. Exercise, air filters, time spent in the forest and at the ocean, and early morning sunlight are important.

➝ Make a point to get adequate rest and sleep during a liver cleanse. The liver does some of its most important work while you sleep!

➝ Reducing dietary fat is crucial for liver health and regeneration. Optimum nutrition is the best liver protection. See "COOKING FOR HEALTHY HEALING" by Linda Rector-Page for complete liver cleansing and healing diets.

➝ A target supplement program accelerates liver detoxification. Royal jelly, ascorbate vitamin C crystals, (at a dose of $1/4$ teasp. at a time), and milk thistle seed extract increase cleansing benefits.

➝ Drink six to eight glasses of bottled water every day to encourage maximum flushing of liver tissues.

Do you need a liver cleanse?

Body signals that your liver needs some TLC include great fatigue, unexplained weight gain, depression or melancholy, mental confusion, sluggish elimination system, food and chemical sensitivity, PMS, jaundiced skin and/or liver spots on the skin, repeated nausea, dizziness and dry mouth.

Herbs are excellent support for liver health

Herbal nutrients quickly begin detoxification and accelerate the blood cleansing process; they normalize, tone and regulate liver functions. They restore the exhausted liver functions of fat metabolism, waste treatment, and acid neutralization. Gallbladder and spleen activity are enhanced to integrate with the liver in producing and storing healthy red blood cells and tissue oxygenation.

Give yourself at least a month or longer for a good liver cleanse. Herbs work methodically and carefully on gland and organ restoration. Healing won't take place overnight, but poor digestion and many glandular deficiencies usually benefit right away.

A broad-based liver restorative course might include several types of herbal preparations used at different stages of the program.

A good place to start is with an alkalizing enzyme body wrap. This is a popular "spring cleaning" technique used in Japan in which herbal extracts are infused into a topical gel and applied to the skin. Because the skin is the body's largest organ of ingestion (and egestion), it can quickly absorb nutrients from the transdermal gel. The specific compound below replaces important minerals, stimulates metabolic activity, neutralizes acid wastes and leaves the body with feeling of well-being. By increasing enzyme and systol/diastole activity, it benefits someone with a poor digestive/elimination condition. Short term cosmetic benefits may be seen in clearer skin as body acids are neutralized, and easier bowel movements as foods are better absorbed. Longer term benefits appear as a more relaxed attitude toward problems and a feeling of well being.

An enzyme gel formula might look like this:
BLADDERWRACK, ALFALFA, GINGER, DANDELION RT., SPEARMINT, CAPSICUM, CINNAMON, ALOE VERA GEL; IN A BASE OF OLIVE OIL, GRAPESEED OIL, LECITHIN, ALOE VERA GEL, VEGETABLE GLYCERINE, BEESWAX.

Increased results would be attained by taking a hot digestive broth two to three times during the day of the wrap. The broth formula might look like this:
MISO GRANUALS, DULSE, BARLEY GREEN GRANUALS, TURMERIC, GINGER.

Adding two concentrated "greens" capsules to the program would offer the best benefits for both liver and whole body. Such a capsule might look like this:
SPIRULINA, ALFALFA LF., VEGETABLE ACIDOPHILUS.

After the enzyme wrap, the next step would be a liver flush tea to help release wastes from the liver and surrounding organs. (If you

decide not to do the enzyme wrap, a liver flush tea would be your first step.) Follow the tea part of the cleanse for one week, taking 2 to 3 cups daily. There are two good herbal options for this step:
1) Use 15 **MILK THISTLE SEED EXTRACT** drops in hot water. Milk Thistle contains some of the most potent liver protecting substances known. The components of this herb stimulate protein synthesis, thereby increasing the production of new liver cells to replace damaged old ones.
2) Use a liver flush tea complex such as the one below: **DANDELION RT., WATERCRESS, YELLOW DOCK RT., PAU D'ARCO, HYSSOP, PARSLEY LF., OREGON GRAPE RT., RED SAGE, LICORICE, MILK THISTLE SD., HIBISCUS FLWR.**

Add a liver cleansing and support capsule combination the second week of your cleanse. Take 3 to 6 capsules daily for three more weeks along with the tea. An effective formula might look like this: **BEET RT., MILK THISTLE SD., OREGON GRAPE RT., DANDELION RT., WILD YAM, YELLOW DOCK RT., GINKGO BILOBA, WILD CHERRY BARK, LICORICE, GOTU KOLA, GINGER, BARBERRY BARK, CHOLINE 15MG, INOSITOL 15MG.**

You will get the best results by following your liver cleanse with an alkalizing diet for a month. This helps restore your new, clean liver to top performance. Fresh foods should form the mainstay, about 60%, of the diet. Protein should come primarily from vegetable sources such as whole grains, soy foods, and beans. The diet should be dairy, alcohol and caffeine free. All saturated fats should be avoided.
Take a brisk walk every day to cleanse the lungs, increase circulation, and oxygenate the blood. Stretching exercises are particularly helpful to liver tissue tone.
Beneficial herbs and supplements during liver rebuilding include:
  ☞ A daily teaspoon of royal jelly
  ☞ Chlorella or spirulina, or a green drink such as the one on page 7, twice a week.
  ☞ Beta-carotene 100,000IU daily with ascorbate vitamin C 3000mg. daily, and vitamin E 400IU daily for anti-infective and anti-oxidant activity.

An ongoing diet for liver health should be lacto-vegetarian, low fat, and rich in vegetable proteins and vitamin C foods for good iron absorption.

BOWEL & COLON CLEANSING

The colon and bowel are the depository for all waste material after nutrients have been extracted and processed to the bloodstream. It is hardly any wonder that up to 90% of all diseases generate from an unclean colon. Unless eliminated regularly, decaying food ferments and forms gases and second generation toxins. The colon becomes a breeding ground for putrefactive bacteria, viruses, parasites, and pathogenic microbes. While the body can tolerate a certain level of contamination, when that individual level is reached, and immune defenses are low, toxic overload causes illness.

Elements causing colon toxicity come from three basic areas:
1) **synthetic chemicals in food and environmental pollutants that range from relatively harmless to dangerous.**
A clean, strong system can metabolize and excrete many of these, but when the body is weak or constipated, they are stored as unusable substances. As more and different chemicals enter the body they tend to interreact with those that are already there, forming mutant, second generation chemicals far more harmful than the originals. Evidence in recent years has shown that most bowel cancer is caused by environmental agents.
2) **overload of body wastes and metabolic byproducts that are not excreted properly.**
These wastes can become a breeding ground for parasite infestation. A nationwide survey reveals that **one in every six people studied** has parasites living somewhere in the body.
3) **slowed elimination time.**
Slow bowel transit time allows waste materials to ferment, become rancid, and then recirculate through the body as toxic substances. Ideally, one should eliminate as often as a meal is taken in. Bowel transit time should be approximately twelve hours.

The most common signals of toxic bowel overload are poor digestion and food assimilation, reduced immune response, fatigue, coated tongue, bad breath and body odor, mental dullness, sallow skin.

A high fiber, whole foods diet is important to both cure and prevent waste elimination problems. Even a gentle, gradual change from low fiber, low residue foods helps almost immediately. In fact, graduated change is better than a sudden, drastic about-face, especially when the colon area is painful or inflamed.

The protective level of fiber in the diet is easily measured:
✔ the stool should be light enough to float.
✔ bowel movements should be regular, daily and effortless.
✔ the stool should be almost odorless, signalling increased transit time in the bowel.
✔ there should be no gas or flatulence.

A colonic irrigation is a good way to start a bowel cleanse. Grapefruit seed extract is very effective, especially if there is colon toxicity along with constipation. (Dilute to 15 to 20 drops in a gallon of water.) Take a catnip enema once a week to keep cleansing well. Note: Enemas may be given to children and infants. Use smaller amounts according to size and age. Allow water to enter very slowly, and allow them to expel when they wish.

Herbal combinations provide cleansing, tonifying activity to cleanse efficiently and gently.
The long history of herbal effectiveness for colon and bowel cleansing allows you to choose a formula for your own specific needs.

The following compound encourages evacuation of the bowels by normal peristalsis. Copious amounts of waste are usually released with this formula. It also tonifies and strengthens the entire elimination system. If taken on a three to six month program to rebuild as well as cleanse the bowel area, this remarkable formula can work in three stages. After current waste is released, hard fecal encrustations are loosened, and cellular acids and wastes are passsed; then the herbs begin a toning action for the bowel walls to promote healing of old lesions and elasticizing of flaccid diverticula, so that regular peristalsis can be restored. This combination may be used successfully for both short and long term advantages, and often works when nothing else has been effective.
BUTTERNUT BARK, CASCARA SAGRADA, TURKEY RHUBARB, PSYLLIUM HUSKS, BARBERRY BK., FENNEL SD., LICORICE, GINGER, IRISH MOSS, CAPSICUM.

This capsule compound provides a mild, gentle cleansing for the bowel when there is irritable bowel soreness, colitis inflammation, or diverticular disease. Demulcent herbs are included to soothe and calm painful spasms, while tonifying herbs encourage elasticity of the bowel muscle.
PEPPERMINT, ALOE VERA, SLIPPERY ELM, MARSHMALLOW RT., PAU D'ARCO, WILD YAM, LOBELIA, GINGER.

🌸 This fiber mix provides easy-to-take organic food fiber necessary to regulate and maintain peristalsis. It is a blend of nature's most complete plant fibers to keep the system clean and healthy. A heaping teaspoon, or four capsules in juice or water at night offer enough soluble fiber for regularity in the morning.
ORGANIC OAT BRAN and FLAX SEED, PSYLLIUM HUSK, GUAR GUM, VEGETABLE ACIDOPHILUS, APPLE PECTIN, ACEROLA CHERRY FIBER, FENNEL SEED, GRAPEFRUIT SEED EXTRACT (as a preservative).

🌸 The following formula is beneficial when a simple herbal laxative is desired, to quickly relieve constipation or to evacuate the bowels before a fast or cleanse. Its nutrients are quick working to temporarily increase systol/diastole activity in the colon and bowel. It should only be used on a limited basis so that the body is assured of doing its own work.
SENNA LF. EXT., FENNEL SEED, PAPAYA LF., PEPPERMINT, GINGER, LEMON BALM, PARSLEY LF., HIBISCUS, CALENDULA.

After the initial cleansing program, the second part of a colon health system is rebuilding healthy tissue and body energy. This stage takes 1 to 2 months for best results. It emphasizes high fiber through fresh vegetables and fruits, cultured foods for increased assimilation and enzyme production, and alkalizing foods to prevent irritation while healing. Avoid refined foods, saturated fats or oils, fried foods, meats, caffeine or other acid/mucous forming foods, such as pasteurized dairy products.
See "COOKING FOR HEALTHY HEALING" by Linda Rector-Page for complete diet and supplement programs for colon cleansing.

Constipation is usually a chronic problem, and while body cleansing progress can be felt fairly quickly with a diet change, it takes from three to six months to rebuild bowel and colon elasticity with good systol/diastole action. Colon cleansing isn't an easy route, but the rewards of a regular, energetic life are worth it.

A good cleanse puts you back in fighting trim!

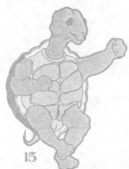

BLADDER & KIDNEY CLEANSING

If you have chronic lower back pain, irritated urination, frequent un-explained chills, fever, or nausea, and unusual fluid retention, you may be feeling the inflammation of a kidney infection. A gentle, nat-ural, kidney cleansing course might be just the thing to keep you from getting a full-blown, painful bladder infection.

The kidneys are largely responsible for the elimination of waste products from protein breakdown (such as urea and ammonia). Concentrated protein wastes can cause chronic inflammation of the kidney filtering tissues (nephritis), and can overload the bloodstream with toxins, causing uremia. Kidney health is the reason most natu-ropaths recommend drinking 6 to 8 glasses of cleansing fluids every day, and limiting animal protein intake.

A kidney cleanse is simple, can be done nutritionally, and is well-supported by herbal remedies. The kidneys are such an integral part of all waste elimination/body purification processes, that a three day cleanse can often clear out toxic infection.

&. Each morning take 2 TBS. cider vinegar or lemon juice in wa-ter. Take **one each** of the following juices each day of the cleanse:

- ➝ carrot/beet/cucumber
- ➝ unsweetened cranberry
- ➝ a mixed vegetable juice
- ➝ a green drink such as the one on page 7
- ➝ **and** drink 6 **extra** glasses of bottled water a day.

&. Eat simply prepared, low salt, low protein, vegetarian foods with 75% in fresh produce. (This type of diet should also be fol-lowed for the two weeks after your cleanse for best results.)

&. After the three days, add sea foods and sea vegetables, whole grains and vegetable proteins. Continue with a morning green drink or the following green tea cleanser for the rest of the month:

&. Kidney healing foods include garlic and onions, papayas, bana-nas, watermelon, sprouts, leafy greens and cucumbers. Take some of these frequently during the rest of the month:
BANCHA LEAF, KUKICHA TWIG, BURDOCK RT., GOTU KOLA, FO-TI, HAWTHORN BERRIES, ORANGE PEEL, CINNAMON.

&. Avoid heavy starches, red and prepared meats, dairy products (except yogurt or kefir), refined, salty, fatty and fast foods for at least a month during healing. They all inhibit kidney filtering .

See the "WASTE MANAGEMENT" booklet in this library se-ries by Linda Rector-Page for more information on bladder and kidney cleansing programs.

What About Fasting As A Detoxification Technique?

Think of fasting as a technique that takes your body back to the starting gate, so that you don't run with a dirty engine or drive with the brakes on. One of the world's oldest known therapies, ancient fasting consisted in abstention from all food and drink except water. Although fasts also had religious overtones, the sound healing principles of fasting were well-known - stress was removed from essential organs and body processes so that healing and rebuilding could take place, while non-essential fatty and muscle tissue was used for fuel.

Fasting has been used regularly up to modern times by naturopaths and herbalists as part of a healing course for a wide range of diseases, both physiological and psychological.

Today, fasting is used primarily as a detoxification method because it is one of the quickest ways to increase elimination of wastes and enhance the healing process. The most dramatic modern results are coming from people whose systems have been contaminated by environmental and chemical pollutants.

With years of experience in fasting programs of all types, I am convinced that a moderate 3 to 7 day juice fast is the best way to release toxins from the system. Shorter fasts don't really get to the root of a chronic or major problem. Longer fasts upset body equilibrium more than most people are ready to deal with except in a controlled, clinical situation.

A well-thought-out moderate juice fast can bring great advantages to the body by cleansing it of excess mucous, old fecal matter, trapped cellular, and non-food wastes, and by "cleaning the pipes" of uncirculated systemic sludge such as inorganic mineral deposits.

A few days without solid food can be a refreshing and enlightening experience about your life style. A short fast increases awareness as well as available energy for elimination. Your body becomes easier to "hear". It can tell you what foods and diet are right for your needs, via legitimate cravings such as a desire for protein foods, B vitamin foods or mineral-rich foods, for example.

Like a "cellular phone call", this is natural biofeedback.

Fasting works by self-digestion. During a cleansing fast, the body in its infinite wisdom, will decompose and burn only the substances and tissue that are damaged, diseased or unneeded, such as abscesses, tumors, excess fat deposits, and congestive wastes. Live, fresh foods and juices can literally pick up dead matter from the body and carry it away.

Even a relatively short fast accelerates elimination from the liver, kidneys, lungs and skin, sometimes causing dramatic body changes as accumulated wastes are expelled. You will be very aware of this phenomenon if you experience the short period of headaches, fatigue, body odor, bad breath, diarrhea or mouth sores that commonly accompany accelerated elimination. Most people encountering these reactions realize that their bodies have thrown off serious toxins because their digestion and many obvious organ functions usually improve right away. A fasting cleanse also helps release hormone secretions that stimulate the immune system.

After a fast, the body starts rebalancing and energy levels begin to rise - physically, psychologically and sexually. Most people notice that creativity begins to expand. Outlook and attitude have changed because actual cell make-up has changed.
You feel like a "different person" - and, of course, you are.

Cleansing The Body Of Congestive Mucous
The following diet is an effective example of a 3 to 7 day liquid fast for detoxification. Elimination will begin as soon as the first meal is missed. Use organically grown fresh fruits and vegetables for all juices if possible.

Have a small fresh salad the night before beginning a liquid fast, with plenty of intestinal "sweepers and scourers", such as beets, celery, cabbage, broccoli, parsley, carrots, etc.

The night before your fast: mash several garlic cloves and a large slice of onion in a bowl. Stir in 3 TBS. of honey. Cover, and let macerate for 24 hours, then remove garlic and onion and take only the honey/syrup infusion - 1 teaspoon, 3 times daily.
On rising: take a glass of fresh-squeezed lemon juice and water, (add 1 TB. maple syrup if desired).
Breakfast: take a glass of grapefruit juice if the system is over-acid; or cranberry/apple or pineapple juice.

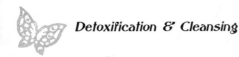
Mid-morning: have a cup of herb tea, such as Japanese green tea, dandelion leaf, or wild cherry bark;
or a tea specifically blended to clear mucous congestion, such as the herbal expectorant below:
MULLEIN LF., PLEURISY RT., LICORICE, ROSEHIPS, MARSHMAL-LOW RT., EPHEDRA EXT., FENNEL, PEPPERMINT, CALENDULA, GINGER, BONESET.
Lunch: take a glass of carrot juice, or mixed vegetable juice.
Mid-afternoon: have a green drink (page 7), or a packet of chlorella or spirulina granules in a glass of water.
Supper: take a glass of apple juice or papaya/pineapple juice.
Before retiring: have a hot broth - place 1 teasp. VEGEX extract paste in 1 cup hot water for relaxation and strength the next day.

↔ During each day of the cleanse, drink 8 glasses of water **in addition** to juices, to thin mucous secretions and aid elimination.
↔ Take 10,000mg. daily of ascorbate vitamin C crystals with bioflavonoids for the first three days. Just dissolve $1/4$ - $1/2$ teasp. in water or juice every hour throughout the day, and take until bowel tolerance is reached, and tissues are flushed.
Take 5,000mg. daily for the next four days.
↔ **For best results,** break your fast with a small fresh salad on the last night of the cleanse.
↔ Begin eating the next day with small simple meals. Have toasted wheat germ or muesli, or whole grain granola for your first morning of solid food, with a little yogurt, apple, or pineapple/coconut juice. Take a small fresh salad for lunch with Italian or lemon/oil dressing. Have a fresh fruit smoothie during the day. Fix a baked potato with butter and a light soup or salad for dinner.

Bodywork Suggestions for a Mucous Cleanse

➤ Take a brisk 1 hour walk each day of the cleanse; breathe deeply to help lungs eliminate mucous.
➤ Take an enema the first and last day of your fasting diet to thoroughly clean out excess mucous.
➤ Take a hot sauna, or long warm baths followed by a brisk rubdown, to stimulate circulation.
You are on your way with a fresh, clean system.

DETOXING FROM ALCOHOL ABUSE

Ground-breaking work is being done today in treating alcohol abuse with nutrition. In the past, two basic treatment methods have been accepted as viable:

1) "talk therapy", based on the assumption that people abuse alcohol because of painful experiences in their past, and that once those events and emotions are dredged up and confronted in group therapy sessions, the desire to escape through alcohol will go away. This type of therapy does not recognize that bio-chemical and neuro-chemical damage done by excess alcohol ingestion cannot be undone by psychological methods alone. It also focuses so heavily on the person's negative reasons and faults for alcohol abuse that it leaves the patient with very little self-worth. Follow-up studies show that only 25% of the people who complete this type of program are sober after a year, **and the success rate decreases from there.**

2) conventional drug therapy, which frequently numbs patients with drugs like Valium or Librium to help ease withdrawal. (Follow-up records are legion with cases of patients who then become addicted to the anti-anxiety drugs.) While most patients acknowledge that withdrawal is easier on these drugs, similar to the effect of 3 or 4 cocktails, they also say that the rest of the program becomes incomprehensible because of the activity of the drugs.

Both methods seek to physically remove the patient from alcohol temptation and from daily life by sequestering him or her in a live-in clinic for a month or more.

Nutritional support treatment recognizes the importance of bio-chemical repair in recovery, assuming that recovery cannot begin until the body begins receiving the essential nutrients it needs. Herbs and amino acids are used to rebalance body chemistry. Necessary and sometimes radical changes are made in diet and lifestyle. Using alcohol as fuel creates multiple nutritional deficiencies of vitamins, minerals, essential fatty acids, amino acids and enzymes. This depletion sets off a chain reaction which results in stress and craving for nutrition. The process is repeated in a futile effort to satisfy increasing need, and addiction eventually occurs.

For the most part nutritional support programs work with clients on an out-patient basis. Although the first results of this new way of treating addictions are just becoming known, early follow-up studies indicate that as many as 75% of patients are still sober after one year.

The normal focus in these programs is first on the physiological imbalances, such as hypoglycemia, that may be causing the alcohol craving. (Over 75% of alcoholics suffer from low blood sugar.)

Since the overwhelming majority of alcohol abusers suffer from malnutrition, patients are given an IV compound of vitamin C as a detoxifier, B vitamins and minerals to help withdrawal symptoms, evening primrose oil as an anti-convulsant, and full spectrum amino acids and glutamine to significantly diminish cravings. They are also given a broad range of nutritional supplements to use at home while they are on the program.

Clients are put on a strict, monitored diet that is sugar, salt, caffeine and nicotine free. (Tobacco leaves are cured with natural sugars, causing intense cravings by hypoglycemics, and latent corn and sugar allergies in others.) The recognition that **allergic** addiction to alcohol is much more common than traditional medicine believes has become a focal point for nutritional treatment programs.

Exercise is part of the plan, to keep body oxygen levels up and blood sugar levels balanced.

Counseling and therapy sessions are also used, generally emphasizing positive actions clients can take to assume control over their lives, rather than seeking out blame for the control that alcohol has over their lives.

Nutritional support is the essential key to establishing a solid nutritional base and revitalizing metabolic deficiencies. Regeneration takes time. It often takes up to a year to detoxify and clear alcohol from the bloodstream.

(See "COOKING FOR HEALTHY HEALING" by Linda Rector-Page for a complete diet, herb and supplement plan to detoxify and rebuild the body from alcohol abuse.)

What can help overcome alcohol craving?

The newest herbal research is showing that the lowly nuisance weed **kudzu** may overcome craving for alcohol. Widely used in China and Japan for centuries to treat alcoholism, kudzu compounds are now available in America. In tests against approved drugs commonly used to blunt the appetite for alcohol, the National Academy of Sciences reported that kudzu worked better.

Although the American experience with kudzu is new, empirical evidence from people taking kudzu capsules for over-consumption of alcohol indicates a definite reduction in alcohol intake.

Kudzu capsules should be taken regularly until craving subsides.

REBUILDING & RESTORING BODY HEALTH

The second part of a good cleansing program is rebuilding healthy tissue and restoring body energy. This stage can usually begin after two to three weeks of waste and toxin elimination.

Effective herbal supplements can make a big difference in the success and rapidity with which the body rebuilds its strength.

Two targets for this stage should include the deep body areas of the glands and organ tissue.

Herbal nutrients can stimulate and nourish exhausted adrenals so that adrenal cortex production and energy can be restored. Adrenal activating formulas have become increasingly popular as continued environmental pollution, lack of quality nutrition, and progressive stress in our lives have caused low adrenal activity. Reduced adrenal function leads to low resistance, chronic fatigue, lethargy, poor circulation, low blood pressure, moodiness and even to dry skin, dull hair, and brittle nails. Effective adrenal activator compounds might look like this:

CAPSULE FORMULA: LICORICE, SARSAPARILLA, BLADDER-WRACK, UVA URSI, ROSEHIPS VIT. C, IRISH MOSS, GINGER, ASTRAGALUS RT., CAPSICUM, PANTOTHENIC ACID 25MG, VIT. B$_6$ 20MG., BETAINE HCL.

EXTRACT FORMULA: LICORICE, SARSAPARILLA, BLADDER-WRACK, IRISH MOSS.

Certain herbs and amino acids that help build healthy muscle and tissue, are synergistic with adrenal stimulating herbs. The formula below is also rich in easily absorbed herbal source minerals. The combination of these strengtheners **taken along with** the adrenal activator formula has proven very effective in rebuilding the body, and should be used for one to two months.

SPIRULINA, BEE POLLEN, ROSEHIPS VIT.C 60MG, ALFALFA LF., FREE FORM AMINO ACID COMPLEX 30MG, BARLEY GRASS, CARROT CALCIUM CRYSTALS, HAWTHORN LF. FLWR. & BRY., SIBERIAN GINSENG, SARSAPARILLA, RED RASPBERRY LF., KELP, WILD CHERRY BK., CHLORELLA, GOLDENSEAL RT., MULLEIN LF., ZINC GLU. 4MG.

A broad spectrum herbal gland balancing formula can nourish, regulate and extend gland and cell life. The one below is for long term rebuilding and should be used for two to three months for best results in energy return and gland vitality.

SARSAPARILLA, SIBERIAN GINSENG, IRISH MOSS, LICORICE, FO-TI, DONG QUAI, BLACK COHOSH, GOTU KOLA, SAW PALMETTO, ALFALFA, KELP, GINGER, SPIRULINA, L-GLUTAMINE 10MG.

The herbs in the next formula act as a haemoglobin builder. They aid in the absorption of iron and other minerals by the glands and organs. The formula encourages increased spleen and liver activity as well as red blood cell production for correction of anemic conditions and symptoms. Ssince a healthy spleen releases oxgenated blood to the body and brain, these herbs also promote mental clarity and resistance to disease.
ALFALFA, BEET RT., DANDELION RT. & LF., PARSLEY RT., YELLOW DOCK, BURDOCK RT., SEBERIAN GINSENG, NETTLES, DULSE, CAPSICUM, HEARTSEASE, BILBERRY.

Naturally-occurring, absorbable potassium is needed as a supplement to revitalize metabolic activity. The healing and rebuilding activity of potassium, calcium and iodine-rich herbs and sea vegetables have made this herbal "K" formula an effective prevention/ wellness formula.
NORWEGIAN KELP, DULSE, BARLEY GRASS POWDER, SPIRULINA, DANDELION RT., WATERCRESS, ALFALFA, PARSLEY RT. & LF., GLUTAMINE-25MG.

Mineral rich herbs are specifics for strong body building blocks. They can provide a regular, daily way to get absorbable minerals, silica and iodine. As the herbal minerals accumulate in the body, a noticeable improvement may be seen in hair, skin and nail health. An effective herbal mineral formula might look like this:
NETTLES, IRISH MOSS, BARLEY GRASS, WATERCRESS, ALFALFA, YELLOW DOCK, KELP, PARSLEY RT., BORAGE SD., PARSLEY LF., DANDELION RT. & LF., DULSE, L-GLUTAMINE 10MG.

New studies on ginseng, cleansing & revitalization....
Ginseng is an excellent first line choice to revitalize the system after a cleansing program. A ginseng blend from around the world can offer a wide range of regenerative activity.

↝ Recognized in China for over 5000 years as a broad spectrum restorative herb, ginseng is now accepted world-wide for its strengthening, revitalizing ability to interact with the human body. Modern clinical research is verifying these attributes and adding new specific applications for ginseng.

↝ An early eighties study in Russia showed ginseng's ability to regulate blood-sugar functions and body acid/alkaline balance. An even more recent success study has involved the therapeutic activity of concentrated ginsenosides on recurrent viral infections and syndromes, such as those occurring in AIDS and other immune deficient diseases.

⇝ Tests in Korea indicate that ginseng strongly inhibits gastric ulcer damage - especially from damage caused by alcohol. Only the whole plant was effective in these tests, not the isolated saponins.

⇝ Studies in both Russia and China are concentraing on ginseng's powerful intercellular anti-oxidant substances, particularly in regard to its anti-aging capabilities, free radical neutralization and immune enhancement.

⇝ Cosmetic companies in both Japan and the U.S. are currently showing successful results for ginseng in a variety of uses from sun and UV protection, to skin aging and wrinkle deterrence.
A purifying, restorative ginseng tea might look like this:
PRINCE GINSENG, KIRIN GINSENG, AMERICAN GINSENG - ARALIA, BRAZILIAN GINSENG - SUMA, SIBERIAN GINSENG - ELUTHERO, TIENCHI GINSENG, PAU D'ARCO, ECHINACEA ANGUSTIFOLIA, ECHINACEA PURPUREA, REISHI MUSHROOMS, ASTRAGALUS RT., ST. JOHN'S WORT, MA HUANG, FENNEL SD.

MAINTAINING A HEALTHY SYSTEM

The final part of a cleansing program is keeping the body clean and toxin-free - very important after all the hard work of detoxification. Modifying lifestyle habits to include high quality nutrition from both food and supplement sources is the key to a strong, resistant body.

The following formula is an herbal whole body tonic. The heavyweights of the herbal kingdom are all included to rebuild tissue, strengthen muscle, maintain stamina and body tone, and enhance immunity. It is a "feel great" compound that may be used in a regular daily optimum nutrition program.
BEE POLLEN, SIBERIAN GINSENG, GOTU KOLA, SARSAPARILLA, LICORICE, ALFALFA, SPIRULINA, RICE PROTEIN, SUMA, SCHIZANDRA, WILD CHERRY BK., BLACK COHOSH, KELP, AMERICAN GINSENG, GOLDENSEAL RT., BARLEY GRASS PWD., NUTRITIONAL YEAST, GINKGO BILOBA, HAWTHORN LF. FLWR. & BRY., CAPSICUM, CHOLINE 10MG, ZINC GLUCONATE 10MG.

About Herbs and How They Work

What are herbs?

Herbs are concentrated foods, edible plants that are safe to take as foods, but are also rich in nutrients that can stimulate the body's healing force, and balance and regulate the human system.

1) Herbs can nourish us, especially with minerals, bolstering deficiencies from poor soil and environment.

2) Herbs can stimulate the body's healing processes by working with the system as body balancers.

Herbal combinations are not addictive or habit-forming, but they are powerful nutritional agents that should be used with common sense and care. Balance is the key to using herbal nutrients for healing. It takes a little more attention and personal responsibility than mindlessly taking a prescription drug. The results are worth it for long term health.

Even though herbs are concentrated, they are whole - not partitioned or isolated substances like drugs. Many drugs use plant isolates and concentrates, but herbs are not drugs. When dealing with chronic long standing problems, I believe the value of herbs lies in their wholeness, not in their concentration. You should not expect the same kind of activity or response that you experience from a chemically formed compound. Drugs treat the symptoms of a problem, so you generally have to take more and more of a drug to get the same effect. It is usually wise to take herbs in descending strength, always asking your body to pick up more and more of its own work.

How do herbs work?

Herbs are foundation support nutrients, working through the glands, nourishing the body's deepest elements, such as the brain, the glands and hormone secretions. Results will seem to take much longer. This is because herbs are working at the deepest levels of body balance and chemistry. **They work at the cause of the problem.** The effects are much more permanent.

However, even with slow steady action, most people feel improvement from herbal treatment in three to six days. Chronic, long standing problems will take longer. The standard rule of thumb is one month of healing for every year you have had the problem.

Herbs do not work like drugs or even like vitamins, where excess amounts flush through the body. Herbs work through the body's enzyme activity, combining with you in the same way that food does. (You are what you eat.) Herbs also contain food enzymes themselves. Their nutritional elements accumulate in the body.

I am always being asked to formulate an herbal maintenance multiple, but I don't think this would serve people well. Taking the same herbs all the time would be like eating the same foods all the time. It would lead to imbalanced nutrition from nutrients that were not in those foods.
Multiple vitamins also work best when strengthening a weak or deficient system. They are not a substitute for a balanced diet.

Herbs work better in combination than they do singly. There are several reasons for this.
1) Each formula compound contains two to five primary agent herbs that are part of the blend for specific purposes. Since all body parts, and most disease symptoms, are interrelated, it is wise to have herbs which can affect each part of the problem.
2) Body balance is encouraged by a combination of herbal nutrients, rather than a large supply of one or two focused properties. A combination gently stimulates the body as a whole.
3) A combination allows inclusion of herbs that can work at different stages of need.
4) A combination of several herbs with similar properties can increase the latitude of effectiveness, not only through a wider range of activity, but also reinforcing herbs that were picked too late or too early, or grew in adverse weather conditions.
5) No two people, or their bodies, are alike. Good response is better insured by a combination of herbs.
6) Finally, some very potent and complex herbs, such as capsicum, lobelia, sassafras, mandrake, tansy, canada snake root, wormwood, woodruff, poke root, and rue are beneficial in small amounts and as catalysts, but should not be used alone.

For more information, see "How To Be Your Own Herbal Pharmacist", a book that clearly shows people how to make and use herbal compounds for themselves, rather than to just use single herbs.

What might I experience during herbal therapy?

1) Occasionally you might experience a mild allergy type reaction as might occur in response to a food. In almost every case, this is not due to the herb itself, but to the chemicals or pesticides used in

the growing or storing process; or because incompatible herbs might have been used together; or just an individual adverse reaction. The key to avoiding adverse reactions is moderation. Anything taken to excess can cause a negative side effect. Use common sense sense when taking herbs as foods or medicines.

2) As with other natural healing programs, you might experience a healing crisis during herbal treatment. This is the "law of cure" and simply means that you will seem to get worse before you get better, as the body goes through a cleansing process to eliminate toxins. Most of us can recognize this as the headache, slight nausea and weakness we feel during a cleansing fast. If there is too much discomfort, simply pace back the herbal treatment to a more comfortable level, and let it take a little longer.

How can I take herbs safely for the best results?

1) Herbs are plants for problems. Therapeutic herbs work best when used on an as-needed basis. **Herbal formulas can be quite specific for a need. Take the formula for your condition at the right time - not all the time - for best results.**
Also, rotating and alternating herbal combinations according to your health goals will allow the body to remain most responsive to their effects.

Like the rest of the natural universe with its 6 day cycle and day of rest, herbs seem to work better with the body when taken for six days in a row, with a rest on the seventh day.

----

2) Take herbs in descending strength, and rest on the seventh day each week. Start with greater amounts at the beginning of your program to build a good healing base; this starts the body's vital balancing force more quickly. As you observe your health returning, fewer and fewer of the large initial doses should be taken. At the end of the program you should be taking maintenance dosage for prevention.
For most people, they realize an herbal treatment has done its job when they forget to take it.

3) It is better to take only one or two herbal combinations at the same time. Choose the treatment that addresses your worst problem first. One of the bonuses of a natural healing program is the discovery that other problems were really complications of the worst one. They will often take care of themselves.

4) Give herbs time to work. Especially with severe, immune deficient, degenerative diseases, it takes a great deal of time to rebuild health. Patience is not an American virtue, but it is important not to add more, except under a qualified practitioner's care, even when your program is working and you can see improvement. We have found over and over again that trying to speed up benefits often only aggravates symptoms and brings worse results. Moderate amounts are excellent, mega-doses are not.
This is because the immune system is a very fragile entity, and can be overwhelmed instead of stimulated. A strong, virulent virus can even be nourished and mutate through supplementation instead of arrested by it. Give your self more time and gentler treatment. Like most other things in life, it ain't just what you do, it's also the way that you do it.

5) Herbs should not be taken like vitamins, i.e. as maintenance to shore up nutrient deficiencies. Except for some food grown vitamins, vitamins are partitioned substances. They don't combine with the body the way herbs do. Excesses are normally flushed through the system if they are not needed.
Herbs combine with the body through it's enzyme activity.

Are herbs safe for children?
Herbs are generally very safe for children. Herb dosage for children (and adults) should be based on body weight:

Child dosage is as follows:
$1/2$ dose for children 10-14 years
$1/3$ dose for children 6-10 years
$1/4$ dose for children 2-6 years
$1/8$ dose for infants and babies

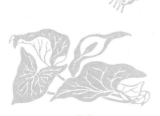

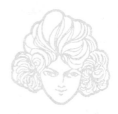

Booklets in the Library Series

Each of Dr. Page's written papers are thoroughly researched - through empirical observation as well as from internationally documented evidence. Studies are ongoing and updated. If you desire reference material, send a self-addressed, stamped envelope with your request to Healthy Healing Publications, 16060 Via Este, Sonora, Ca., 95370.

A Last Word About Herbs

Science can only quantify, isolate, and assay to understand. Herbs respond to these methods, but they are so much more than a scientific breakdown. God shows his face a little in herbs. Like mankind, herbs also have an ineffable quality. Fortunately for mankind, our bodies know how to use herbs without our brains having to know why.

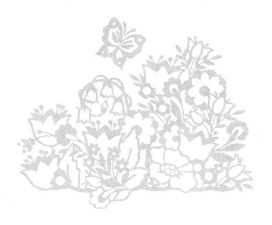

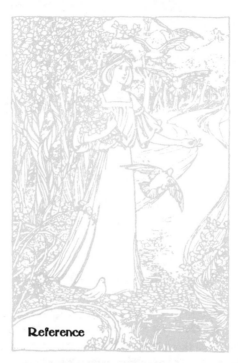

Reference

BIBLIOGRAPHY

Deininger, R. "Amarum-Bitter Herbs: Common Bitter Principle Remedies and Their Action." **Krankenpflege.** 29 (3) (1975): 99-100.

Foster, Steven. **Milk Thistle.** Austin: American Botanical Council, 1991.

Hahn, G., et al. "On the Pharmacology and Toxicology of Silymarin, An Anti-Hepatotoxic Active Principle for Silybum Marianum." **Arzneimittelforschung.** 18 (6) (1968): 698-704.

Hendler, Sheldon Saul, M.D., Ph.D. **The Purification Prescription.** New York: William Morrow and Co., Inc., 1991.

Hikino, H., et al. "Antihepatotoxic Actions of Flavonolignans from Silybum Marianum Fruits." **Planta Medica.** 50 (1984): 248-50

Holmes, Peter. **The Energetics of Western Herbs.** Berkeley: NatTrop Publishing, 1993.

Poser, G. "Experience in the Treatment of Chronic Hepatopathies with Silymarin." **Arzneimittelforschung.** 21 (8) (1971): 1209-12

Quillin, Patrick, Ph.D., R.D. **Healing Nutrients.** Chicago: Contemporary Books, 1987.

Rogers, Sherry A., M.D. **Tired or Toxic? A Blueprint for Health.** N.p.: Prestige NY, 1990.

Saifer, Phyllis. **Detox.** Los Angeles: Jeremy Tarcher, 1984.

Salaman, Maureen and James Scheer. **Foods That Heal.** Menlo Park: Statford Publications, 1989.

Salmi, H.A., and S. Sarna. "Effect of Silymarin on Chemical, Functional, and Morphological Alterations of the Liver: A Double-Blind Controlled Study." **Scand. J. Gastroenterol.** 17 (1982): 517-21.

Shannon, Sarah. **Diet for the Atomic Age.** Garden City Park: Avery Publishing Group, 1987.

Vander, Arthur J., M.D. **Nutrition, Stress and Toxic Chemicals.** N.p.: University of Michigan Press, 1981.

Vogel, G., et al. "Studies on Pharmacodynamics, Site and Mechanism of Action of Silymarin, the Antihepatotoxic Principle from Silybum Marianum." **Arzneimittelforschung,** 25 (1975): 179-85.

Wagner, H. "Plant Constituents with Antihepatotoxic Activity." **Natural Products as Medicinal Agents.** Stuttgart: Hippokrates-Verlag, 1981.

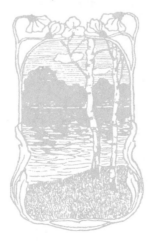

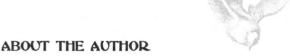

ABOUT THE AUTHOR

Linda Rector-Page has been working with nutrition and herbal medicinals both professionally and as a personal life style choice, since the early seventies. She is a certified Doctor of Naturopathy and Ph.D., with extensive experience in formulating and testing herbal combinations. She received a Doctor of Naturopathy degree from the Clayton School of Holistic Healing in 1988, and a Ph.D. in Nutritional Therapy from the American Holistic College of Nutrition in 1989. She is a member of both the American and California Naturopathic Medical Associations.

She opened and operated the "Rainbow Kitchen", a natural foods restaurant, worked as an employee, and then became a working partner in The Country Store Natural Foods store. She has written three successful books in the nutritional healing field, and is founder/developer of Crystal Star Herbal Nutrition.

Ongoing contact with many manufacturers and distributors of natural products has proved very beneficial in writing her book, "HEALTHY HEALING", now in its ninth edition. In addition, Crystal Star Herbal Nutrition products, which are formulated by Linda, are carried by over two thousand natural food stores nationwide. Feedback from these direct consumer sources provides up-to-the–minute contact with the needs, desires and results being experienced by people taking more responsibility for their own health. Much of the lifestyle information and empirical observation detailed in her books comes from this direct experience. This knowledge is then translated into lifestyle therapies, and recorded in every "HEALTHY HEALING" edition.

"COOKING FOR HEALTHY HEALING", now in its second revised edition, is a companion to "HEALTHY HEALING". It draws on both the recipes from the Rainbow Kitchen and the more defined healthy lifestyle diets that she has developed from healing results since then. The book contains thirty-three separate diet programs, and over 900 healthy recipes. Every recipe has been taste-tested and time-tested as a part of each recommended diet, so that the suggested healing program can be maintained easily and deliciously with the highest nutrition.

In her latest book, "HOW TO BE YOUR OWN HERBAL PHARMACIST", Linda addesses the rising appeal of herbs and herbal healing in America. Many people have expressed interest in clearly understanding herbal formulation knowledge for themselves. This book is designed for those wishing to take more definitive responsibility for their health through individually developed herbal combinations.

Published by Healthy Healing Publications, 1994.